STAGE 3 KIDNEY DISEASE DIET COOKBOOK FOR SENIORS

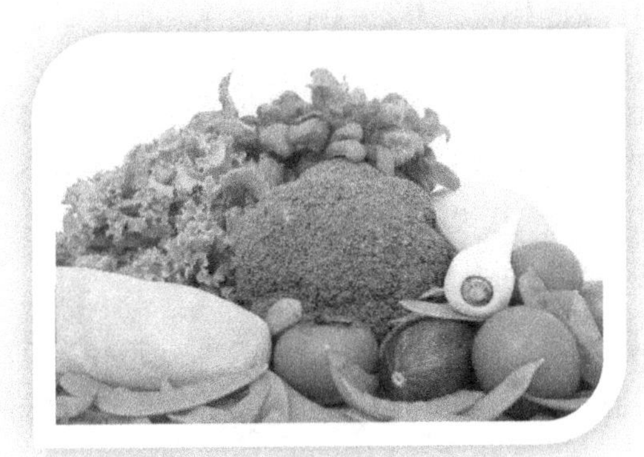

The Ultimate Nutrition Guide With Low Sodium, Low Potassium, and Low Phosphorus Kidney friendly Recipes for older people

Dr. Mary D. Cook

TABLE OF CONTENTS

INTRODUCTION

In the realm of real-life triumphs over adversity, let me share with you the inspiring journey of Mr. Harold Thompson, a resilient soul who faced the challenge of stage 3 kidney disease head-on.

As a seasoned nutritionist, I've witnessed the transformative power of a well-crafted diet, and Mr. Thompson's story is a testament to the profound impact it can have on one's health.

Mr. Thompson a spry gentleman in his late sixties, He had spent a considerable portion of his life blissfully unaware of the silent threat lurking within — stage 3 kidney disease. Upon receiving this diagnosis, he found himself at a crossroads, unsure of how to navigate the complexities of his newfound health predicament.

In our initial meeting, Mr. Thompson's eyes reflected a mixture of determination and uncertainty.

Together, we embarked on a personalized journey, crafting a dietary plan tailored to his unique needs, a plan that would eventually become the linchpin of his triumphant tale.

Gone were the days of indiscriminate indulgence. Instead, we embraced the notion that food could be both medicine and nourishment. A symphony of low-sodium, low-phosphorus, and low-potassium delights graced Mr. Thompson's plate, each carefully chosen to support his kidneys and stave off the progression of his condition.

The first weeks were a delicate dance of adaptation. Yet, as Mr. Thompson immersed himself in this new culinary narrative, the subtle alchemy of wholesome ingredients began to work its magic. Leafy greens, lean proteins, and a rainbow of vegetables became the protagonists of his daily sustenance, gradually altering the trajectory of his health.

As the seasons changed, so did Mr. Thompson's lab results.

The markers that once stood as harbingers of kidney distress now whispered tales of improvement. A testament to the power of mindful nutrition and the body's remarkable capacity to heal.

We celebrated small victories — stabilized blood pressure, improved kidney function, and a newfound vitality that echoed in Mr. Thompson's laughter, which now resonated with a vigor that belied his years.

Mr. Thompson's story is not one of fantasy but of triumph over adversity, where the protagonist, armed with the right diet, rewrote the narrative of his health. His journey teaches us that the script of our well-being is not set in stone. With dedication, guidance, and the right nourishment, we can script a future of resilience and vitality, no matter our age or the challenges we face.

So, as you delve into the pages of nutritional wisdom, remember the tale of Mr. Harold Thompson — a living testament to the transformative power of a diet designed with care and intention.

A story that speaks to the boundless potential within each of us to rewrite the narrative of our health.

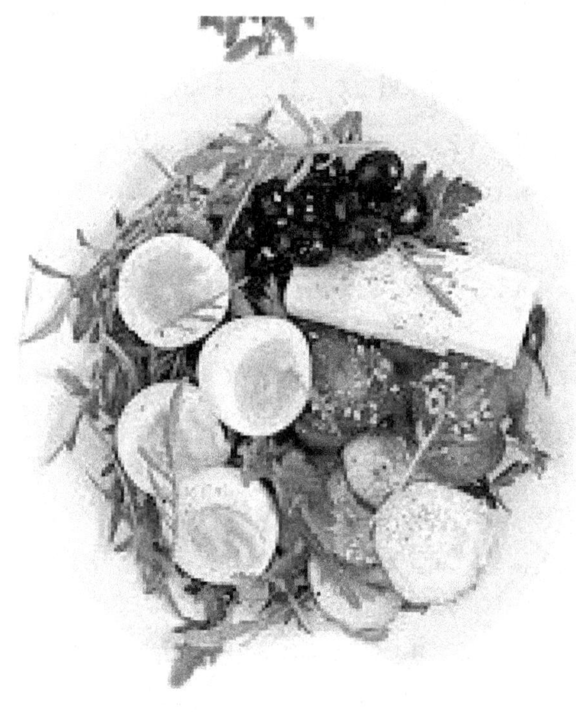

CHAPTER 1

Understanding Stage 3 Kidney Disease

The kidneys, those unassuming bean-shaped marvels, play a vital role in our lives. They filter our blood, removing waste and toxins, balancing fluids and electrolytes, and helping regulate blood pressure. But sometimes, these tireless organs face challenges, leading to a condition known as chronic kidney disease (CKD). Within this spectrum, Stage 3 CKD signifies a crucial juncture, a time for both concern and proactive action.

A Glimpse Inside the Filtering Factory:

Imagine your kidneys as a complex filtration system. They are comprised of millions of tiny nephrons, each acting as a miniature filter. Blood flows through these nephrons, and essential nutrients are reabsorbed into the bloodstream, while waste products and excess fluids are expelled as urine. This intricate process keeps our internal environment stable and healthy.

The Stage 3 Scenario:

In Stage 3 CKD, the nephrons begin to lose their filtering capacity. This doesn't mean they stop working altogether, but their efficiency diminishes. Think of it like a clogged drainpipe – the flow is slower, and some debris may slip through. As a consequence, waste products can build up in the bloodstream, leading to a cascade of potential complications.

The Symptoms: A Subtle Chorus:

Stage 3 CKD often whispers its arrival. Early symptoms can be subtle and easily mistaken for other conditions. Fatigue, high blood pressure, frequent urination (especially at night), and itching are some common clues.

However, the absence of these symptoms doesn't rule out the disease, making regular checkups and early detection crucial.

The Diagnosis: A Crossroads of Choices:

A diagnosis of Stage 3 CKD can feel daunting. However, it's important to remember that it's not a dead end, but rather a crossroads. This is an opportunity to take control and implement strategies to slow disease progression and improve overall health.

The cornerstones of managing Stage 3 CKD:

Dietary Modifications: A kidney-friendly diet becomes essential. This involves limiting sodium, potassium, and phosphorus, while prioritizing essential nutrients like fiber and protein. Think fresh fruits and vegetables, whole grains, and lean protein sources.

Blood Pressure Control: High blood pressure can accelerate kidney damage.

Medications and lifestyle changes, such as exercise and stress management, can help keep it in check.

Blood Sugar Management: Diabetes and CKD often go hand-in-hand. Controlling blood sugar through medication and lifestyle modifications is crucial for both conditions.

Medications: Specific medications may be prescribed to manage symptoms, protect remaining kidney function, and address complications like anemia or bone disease.

Regular Monitoring: Close follow-up with your healthcare team is vital. Regular blood tests, urine tests, and imaging studies help assess kidney function and adjust treatment plans as needed.

The Power of Proactive Lifestyle:

Beyond medical interventions, proactive lifestyle changes play a significant role in managing Stage 3 CKD. Regular physical activity, stress management techniques like yoga or meditation, and adequate sleep all contribute to overall health and kidney well-being.

Living Well with Stage 3 CKD:

Living with Stage 3 CKD requires adjustments, but it doesn't have to diminish the quality of life. With the right support, information, and proactive management, individuals with Stage 3 CKD can lead full and active lives. It's a journey, not a destination, one where knowledge, empowerment, and a supportive network become your compass and companions.

Remember, Stage 3 CKD is a condition, not a sentence. By understanding the disease, implementing effective management strategies, and embracing a proactive lifestyle, individuals can navigate this crossroads with determination, hope, and a zest for life.

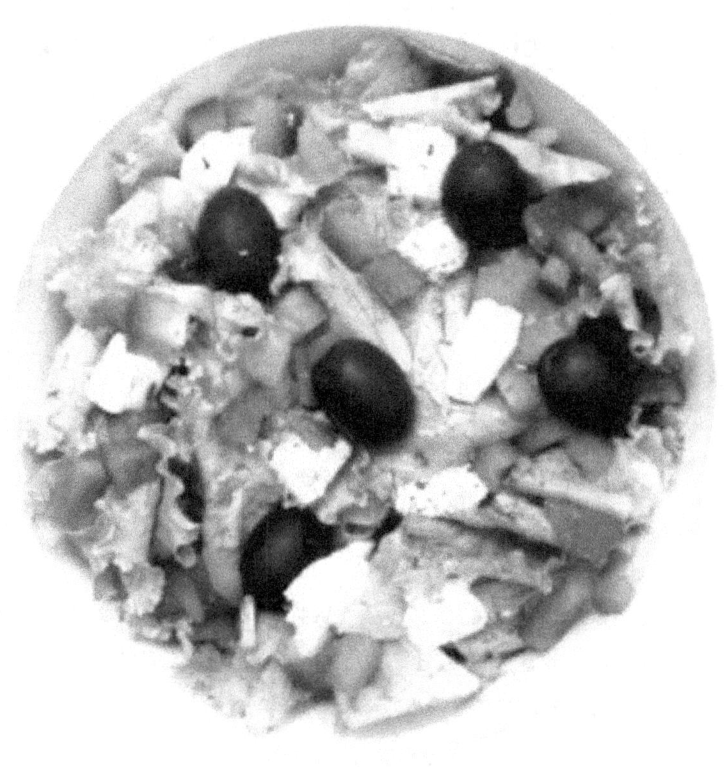

CHAPTER 2

The Core benefits of following kidney disease diet for seniors

Following a kidney disease diet tailored for seniors offers several core benefits that contribute to overall health and well-being. Here are the key advantages:

Blood Pressure Management:

A kidney-friendly diet often emphasizes low sodium intake, which is crucial for managing blood pressure. By reducing sodium, seniors can help regulate blood pressure levels, reducing the strain on their kidneys.

Protein Control:

Seniors with kidney disease may be advised to moderate their protein intake. This helps prevent the buildup of waste products in the blood, easing the workload on the kidneys.

High-quality, low-phosphorus protein sources, such as lean meats and eggs, are typically recommended.

Phosphorus Regulation:

Kidney disease can lead to difficulty in regulating phosphorus levels. A kidney disease diet for seniors often includes foods with lower phosphorus content, such as fruits and vegetables, to prevent complications like bone and cardiovascular issues.

Potassium Balance:

Kidneys play a role in balancing potassium levels in the body. Seniors with kidney disease may need to manage their potassium intake, as imbalances can lead to heart and muscle problems. Choosing low-potassium foods like apples, berries, and cauliflower helps maintain this balance.

Fluid Control:

Proper fluid management is crucial for individuals with kidney disease.

Following a kidney-friendly diet helps seniors control their fluid intake, preventing fluid retention, swelling, and complications related to imbalanced electrolytes.

Improved Nutrient Intake:

A kidney disease diet doesn't mean sacrificing nutrition. It encourages seniors to focus on nutrient-dense foods, ensuring they receive essential vitamins and minerals. This is particularly important for maintaining overall health and supporting the body's immune system.

Heart Health Support:

Many aspects of a kidney disease diet align with heart-healthy eating patterns. By reducing sodium, saturated fats, and cholesterol, seniors can not only support kidney health but also contribute to cardiovascular well-being, reducing the risk of heart-related complications.

Prevention of Malnutrition:

Kidney disease can sometimes lead to malnutrition due to dietary restrictions and loss of appetite. A well-planned kidney disease diet ensures that seniors receive adequate nutrition, preventing deficiencies and supporting energy levels.

Customization to Individual Needs:

One of the strengths of a kidney disease diet is its adaptability. It can be customized based on an individual's specific health needs, stage of kidney disease, and other medical conditions. This tailoring ensures that seniors receive dietary recommendations that are personalized to their unique requirements.

Enhanced Quality of Life:

By adhering to a kidney disease diet, seniors can experience an improvement in their overall quality of life. Managing symptoms, reducing the progression of kidney disease, and promoting general well-being contribute to a more fulfilling and active lifestyle.

The complications of stage 3 kidney disease, if the right diet isn't adopted.

Failure to adopt the right diet in Stage 3 Kidney Disease can lead to several complications, as the kidneys are already compromised in their ability to filter waste products and maintain fluid and electrolyte balance. Here are some potential complications:

1. Progression to Advanced Stages:

Without proper dietary management, Stage 3 Kidney Disease can progress to more advanced stages. The kidneys may further decline in function, increasing the risk of complications associated with more severe kidney impairment.

2. Fluid Retention and Edema:

Inadequate control of sodium and fluid intake can result in fluid retention, leading to swelling (edema) in various parts of the body, such as the hands, legs, and face. This can contribute to increased blood pressure and strain on the heart.

3. Electrolyte Imbalances:

The kidneys play a crucial role in maintaining the balance of electrolytes in the body, including potassium and phosphorus. Failure to regulate these electrolytes through diet can lead to imbalances, causing issues such as muscle weakness, irregular heartbeat, and bone problems.

4. High Blood Pressure:

The kidneys play a significant role in regulating blood pressure. Ineffective management of sodium intake and other dietary factors can contribute to hypertension, further damaging the kidneys and increasing the risk of cardiovascular complications.

5. Anemia:

Inadequate control of phosphorus and other minerals can lead to complications such as renal anemia. The kidneys produce erythropoietin, a hormone essential for red blood cell production.

Dysfunction in this process can result in anemia, leading to fatigue and weakness.

6. Bone Health Issues:

Phosphorus balance is crucial for bone health. If phosphorus levels are not properly controlled through diet, it can lead to the leaching of calcium from the bones, contributing to bone problems such as bone pain and fractures.

7. Compromised Immune System:

Malnutrition and deficiencies in essential nutrients due to an improper diet can weaken the immune system. This makes individuals more susceptible to infections and further complicates the management of kidney disease.

8. Cardiovascular Complications:

Kidney disease is a known risk factor for cardiovascular problems. Inadequate dietary management can exacerbate this risk, leading to conditions such as heart disease and stroke.

9. Gastrointestinal Issues:

Kidney disease can affect the gastrointestinal tract, leading to issues like nausea, vomiting, and poor appetite. Failing to adopt the right diet can exacerbate these symptoms, making it difficult to maintain adequate nutrition.

10. General Fatigue and Weakness:

Complications arising from poor dietary choices can contribute to overall fatigue and weakness. This can significantly impact the quality of life and daily functioning of individuals with Stage 3 Kidney Disease.

Regular monitoring of kidney function and adjustments to the diet are essential components of managing the disease and preventing complications.

Foods to Eat:

1. Low-Phosphorus Fruits and Vegetables:

Emphasize fruits and vegetables with low phosphorus content, such as berries, apples, cucumbers, and bell peppers. These options provide essential vitamins and fiber without overloading on phosphorus.

2. Lean Proteins:

Opt for lean protein sources, including skinless poultry, fish, eggs, and plant-based proteins like tofu and legumes. These choices offer high-quality protein without excessive phosphorus or potassium.

3. Whole Grains:

Choose whole grains like brown rice, quinoa, and whole wheat bread. These provide energy and fiber without contributing to phosphorus buildup.

4. Healthy Fats:

Include sources of healthy fats, such as olive oil, avocados, and nuts. These fats support overall health without negatively impacting kidney function.

5. Low-Sodium Foods:

Select low-sodium alternatives to manage blood pressure. Fresh herbs, spices, and homemade seasonings can add flavor without the need for excessive salt.

6. Calcium-Rich Foods:

Consume moderate amounts of calcium through sources like low-fat dairy (if permitted), fortified plant-based milk, and leafy greens. Adequate calcium helps maintain bone health without overwhelming phosphorus levels.

7. Hydrating Options:

Stay well-hydrated with water, herbal teas, and limited amounts of clear broths.

Proper hydration supports kidney function and helps prevent complications related to fluid retention.

8. Cabbage and Cucumber:

These vegetables are not only low in potassium but also have a diuretic effect, aiding in fluid balance.

Foods to Limit:

1. Red and Processed Meats:

Limit the intake of red and processed meats, as they are high in phosphorus and may contribute to the progression of kidney disease.

2. Dairy Products:

Consume dairy products in moderation, as they contain phosphorus. Choose low-phosphorus options and consider alternatives like almond or rice milk.

3. Processed Foods:

Reduce the consumption of processed and packaged foods, as they often contain hidden sodium, preservatives, and additives that can be detrimental to kidney health.

4. High-Potassium Fruits and Vegetables:

While fruits and vegetables are essential, limit high-potassium choices like bananas, oranges, tomatoes, and potatoes. Instead, use them in moderation.

5. Nuts and Seeds:

Control portions of nuts and seeds due to their phosphorus content. Consider soaking them before consumption to reduce phosphorus levels.

6. Certain Whole Grains:

Limit certain whole grains like bran cereals and whole wheat products, as they can be higher in phosphorus.

Minimize salt intake to control blood pressure. Avoid processed and salty foods, and opt for fresh, whole foods seasoned with herbs and spices.

8. Dark-Colored Sodas:

Limit or avoid dark-colored sodas, as they may contain phosphorus additives that can be harmful to kidney health.

20 healthy smart shopping for a Stage 3 Kidney-Friendly Ingredients:

1. Lean Proteins:

- Skinless poultry (chicken, turkey)
- Fish (salmon, cod, trout)
- Eggs (consider using egg whites)

2. Low-Phosphorus Fruits:

- Berries (strawberries, blueberries, raspberries)
- Apples
- Pineapple

3. Low-Potassium Vegetables:

- Cabbage
- Cauliflower
- Bell peppers

4. Whole Grains:

- Brown rice
- Quinoa
- Whole wheat bread (in moderation)

5. Healthy Fats:

- Olive oil
- Avocados
- Nuts (in controlled portions)

6. Low-Sodium Seasonings:

- Fresh herbs (parsley, cilantro, basil)
- Spices (cumin, turmeric, garlic powder)

7. Low-Phosphorus Dairy Alternatives:

- Almond milk (fortified with calcium)
- Rice milk (calcium-fortified)

8. Hydration Options:

- Bottled water
- Herbal teas (non-caffeinated)
- Low-sodium broths

9. Low-Potassium Pasta Alternatives:

- Pasta made from rice or corn
- Egg noodles (in moderation)

10. Low-Phosphorus Snacks:

- Popcorn (air-popped)
- Rice cakes

11. Fresh Vegetables:

- Zucchini
- Green beans
- Kale (in moderation)

12. Low-Potassium Fruits:

- Cranberries
- Peaches (in moderation)
- Plums

13. Low-Phosphorus Condiments:

- Mustard
- Vinegar
- Lemon juice

14. Low-Potassium Dairy:

- Cream cheese
- Ricotta cheese

15. Low-Phosphorus Dessert Options:

- Angel food cake
- Sherbet

16. Low-Sodium Canned Goods:

- Low-sodium canned beans (rinse them to reduce sodium)
- Low-sodium tomato sauce

17. Low-Phosphorus Grains:

- Couscous
- Bulgur

18. Low-Potassium Salad Greens:

- Iceberg lettuce
- Arugula

19. Low-Phosphorus Meats:

- Ground turkey
- Pork (in moderation)

20. Low-Potassium Sweeteners:

- Honey (in moderation)
- Maple syrup (in moderation)

When shopping for these ingredients, it's essential to check product labels for nutritional information, especially regarding sodium, phosphorus, and potassium content.

Essential Kitchen Tips for Seniors: Simplifying Meal Preparation:

Meal preparation can be a delightful and empowering activity for seniors, contributing not only to nutrition but also to overall well-being. Here are some essential kitchen tips tailored to simplify meal preparation for seniors:

1. Organize Your Kitchen:

Keep commonly used utensils, pots, and pans within easy reach. Organize your kitchen to minimize the need for reaching or bending, reducing strain on joints.

2. Invest in Time-Saving Appliances:

Consider using time-saving appliances like a slow cooker, Instant Pot, or microwave. These tools can make cooking more efficient and less physically demanding.

3. Prep Ingredients in Advance:

Take advantage of times when you have more energy to prepare and store ingredients in advance. Chop vegetables, portion meats, and pre-measure ingredients to streamline the cooking process.

4. Explore Pre-Packaged Healthy Options:

Opt for pre-packaged healthy options, such as pre-cut vegetables, frozen fruits, or pre-cooked proteins. These can significantly reduce preparation time without compromising nutrition.

5. Use Adaptive Kitchen Tools:

Consider using adaptive kitchen tools designed for ease of use.

Items like ergonomic utensils, easy-grip knives, and jar openers can make cooking more accessible for seniors.

6. Implement Simple Cooking Techniques:

Focus on simple cooking techniques that require minimal effort, such as roasting, grilling, or one-pot meals. These methods can enhance flavors without the need for extensive preparation.

7. Plan Simple Menus:

Plan simple and balanced menus. Choose recipes with fewer ingredients and straightforward instructions to make the cooking process more manageable.

8. Embrace Batch Cooking:

Prepare larger quantities of meals and freeze individual portions for later use. This minimizes the frequency of cooking and ensures a readily available supply of nutritious meals.

9. Explore Healthy Convenience Foods:

Incorporate healthy convenience foods like pre-cooked brown rice, canned beans, or low-sodium broths. These items can serve as a base for quick and nutritious meals.

10. Create a Comfortable Cooking Environment:

Ensure that your kitchen is well-lit, and the workspace is comfortable. Consider using non-slip mats to enhance safety and reduce the risk of accidents.

11. Practice Kitchen Safety:

Pay attention to kitchen safety. Use oven mitts, pot holders, and other protective gear to avoid burns. Keep a fire extinguisher within reach for added safety.

12. Opt for One-Step Snacks:

Choose easy one-step snacks, such as fresh fruit, yogurt, or cheese slices. These snacks are not only nutritious but also require minimal preparation.

13. Experiment with Flavorful Herbs and Spices:

Elevate the taste of your meals with flavorful herbs and spices. Experimenting with different combinations can add variety to your diet without complicating the cooking process.

14. Consider Meal Delivery Services:

Explore meal delivery services that offer healthy, pre-prepared options. This can be a convenient solution for days when cooking feels challenging.

15. Delegate Tasks and Share Meals:

If possible, involve family members or friends in meal preparation. Sharing the cooking responsibilities can make the process more enjoyable and efficient.

16. Stay Hydrated:

Don't forget the importance of staying hydrated. Keep water easily accessible in the kitchen to promote regular intake throughout the day.

17. Keep a Well-Stocked Pantry:

Maintain a well-stocked pantry with staples like canned vegetables, whole grains, and low-sodium sauces. This ensures you have the basics on hand for quick and easy meal assembly.

18. Stay Mindful of Portion Sizes:

Be mindful of portion sizes to avoid waste and ensure you're getting the right amount of nutrients. Invest in smaller-sized kitchenware for more accurate measurements.

19. Create a Weekly Meal Plan:

Plan your meals for the week ahead. Having a structured meal plan reduces decision fatigue and makes grocery shopping more efficient.

20. Enjoy the Process:

Finally, savor the process of preparing and enjoying your meals. Cooking can be a pleasurable and therapeutic activity, contributing to a positive mindset and overall well-being.

By implementing these kitchen tips, you can simplify meal preparation, making it a more enjoyable and manageable part of your daily routine.

STAGE 3 KIDNEY FRIENDLY DIETS:

BREAKFASTS THAT NOURISH:

1. Quinoa Breakfast Bowl

Ingredients:

- 1/2 cup cooked quinoa
- 1/4 cup fresh berries
- 1 tablespoon chopped almonds
- 1 teaspoon chia seeds
- 1/2 teaspoon cinnamon
- 1/2 cup almond milk (unsweetened)

Preparation:

1. In a bowl, combine cooked quinoa, fresh berries, chopped almonds, chia seeds, and cinnamon.
2. Pour almond milk over the mixture.
3. Stir gently and enjoy!

Servings: 1 | **Nutritional Value (per serving):** Calories: 250, Protein: 8g, Fiber: 7g, Carbs: 35g, Fat: 9g | Cooking Time: 15 minutes

2. Egg White Vegetable Omelette

Ingredients:

- 2 egg whites
- 1/4 cup diced bell peppers
- 1/4 cup spinach, chopped
- 1 tablespoon diced tomatoes
- 1 teaspoon olive oil
- Salt and pepper to taste

Preparation:

1. Whisk egg whites in a bowl until frothy.
2. In a non-stick pan, sauté bell peppers, spinach, and tomatoes in olive oil.
3. Pour whisked egg whites over the veggies, cook until set, and fold into an omelette.

Servings: 1 | Nutritional Value (per serving): Calories: 150, Protein: 18g, Fiber: 3g, Carbs: 8g, Fat: 5g | Cooking Time: 10 minutes

3. Greek Yogurt Parfait

Ingredients:

- 1/2 cup Greek yogurt (unsweetened)
- 1/4 cup granola (low-sugar)
- 1/4 cup fresh berries
- 1 tablespoon sliced almonds
- 1/2 teaspoon honey (optional)

Preparation:

1. In a glass, layer Greek yogurt, granola, fresh berries, and sliced almonds.
2. Drizzle with honey if desired.

Servings: 1 | Nutritional Value (per serving): Calories: 250, Protein: 15g, Fiber: 5g, Carbs: 25g, Fat: 10g | Preparation Time: 5 minutes

4. Sweet Potato Pancakes

Ingredients:

- 1/2 cup mashed sweet potatoes
- 2 tablespoons oat flour
- 1 egg
- 1/4 teaspoon baking powder
- 1/2 teaspoon cinnamon
- 1/4 cup almond milk (unsweetened)

Preparation:

1. In a bowl, mix mashed sweet potatoes, oat flour, egg, baking powder, and cinnamon.
2. Add almond milk to achieve a pancake batter consistency.
3. Cook spoonfuls of batter on a griddle until golden brown.

Servings: 2 | Nutritional Value (per serving): Calories: 180, Protein: 8g, Fiber: 4g, Carbs: 30g, Fat: 4g | Cooking Time: 15 minutes

5. Chia Seed Pudding with Almond Butter

Ingredients:

- 2 tablespoons chia seeds
- 1/2 cup almond milk (unsweetened)
- 1/2 teaspoon vanilla extract
- 1 tablespoon almond butter
- 1/4 cup sliced strawberries

Preparation:

1. Mix chia seeds, almond milk, and vanilla extract in a jar. Refrigerate overnight.
2. Top with almond butter and sliced strawberries before serving.

Servings: 1 | Nutritional Value (per serving): Calories: 250, Protein: 7g, Fiber: 12g, Carbs: 20g, Fat: 15g | Preparation Time: 5 minutes (plus overnight refrigeration)

6. Spinach and Feta Frittata Muffins

Ingredients:

- 3 eggs
- 1/4 cup feta cheese, crumbled
- 1/2 cup fresh spinach, chopped
- 1/4 cup cherry tomatoes, halved
- Salt and pepper to taste

Preparation:

1. Preheat oven to 350°F (175°C).
2. In a bowl, whisk eggs and mix in feta, spinach, and cherry tomatoes.
3. Pour into greased muffin tin and bake for 15-20 minutes.

Servings: 2 | Nutritional Value (per serving): Calories: 180, Protein: 14g, Fiber: 2g, Carbs: 5g, Fat: 12g | Cooking Time: 20 minutes

7. Cottage Cheese and Pineapple Bowl

Ingredients:

- 1/2 cup low-fat cottage cheese
- 1/2 cup fresh pineapple chunks
- 1 tablespoon shredded coconut
- 1 teaspoon honey (optional)

Preparation:

1. In a bowl, combine cottage cheese and pineapple.
2. Top with shredded coconut and drizzle with honey if desired.

Servings: 1 | Nutritional Value (per serving): Calories: 200, Protein: 15g, Fiber: 2g, Carbs: 25g, Fat: 5g | Preparation Time: 5 minutes

8. Avocado and Smoked Salmon Toast

Ingredients:

- 1 slice whole grain bread
- 1/4 avocado, mashed
- 2 ounces smoked salmon
- Lemon juice and dill for garnish

Preparation:

1. Toast the bread slice.
2. Spread mashed avocado on the toast and top with smoked salmon.
3. Garnish with lemon juice and dill.

Servings: 1 | Nutritional Value (per serving): Calories: 250, Protein: 18g, Fiber: 5g, Carbs: 20g, Fat: 12g | Preparation Time: 10 minutes

9. Oatmeal with Berries and Almond Milk

Ingredients:

- 1/2 cup rolled oats
- 1/2 cup almond milk (unsweetened)
- 1/4 cup mixed berries
- 1 tablespoon chopped almonds
- 1/2 teaspoon cinnamon

Preparation:

1. Cook rolled oats with almond milk on the stovetop.
2. Top with mixed berries, chopped almonds, and a sprinkle of cinnamon.

Servings: 1 | Nutritional Value (per serving): Calories: 220, Protein: 8g, Fiber: 6g, Carbs: 35g, Fat: 7g | Cooking Time: 7 minutes

10. Turkey and Veggie Breakfast Wrap

Ingredients:

- 1 whole wheat tortilla
- 2 ounces turkey breast, sliced
- 1/4 cup sautéed bell peppers and onions
- 1 tablespoon salsa (low-sodium)

Preparation:

1. Warm the tortilla.
2. Layer turkey, sautéed bell peppers and onions, and salsa.
3. Roll up and enjoy.

Servings: 1 | Nutritional Value (per serving): Calories: 230, Protein: 20g, Fiber: 5g, Carbs: 25g, Fat: 8g | Preparation Time: 10 minutes

11. Blueberry Almond Smoothie Bowl

Ingredients:

- 1/2 cup frozen blueberries
- 1/2 banana
- 1/2 cup almond milk (unsweetened)
- 1 tablespoon almond butter
- 2 tablespoons granola (low-sugar)

Preparation:

1. Blend blueberries, banana, almond milk, and almond butter until smooth.
2. Pour into a bowl and top with granola.

Servings: 1 | Nutritional Value (per serving): Calories: 260, Protein: 8g, Fiber: 7g, Carbs: 35g, Fat: 10g | Preparation Time: 5 minutes

12. Mushroom and Herb Scramble

Ingredients:

- 2 eggs
- 1/4 cup mushrooms, sliced
- 1 tablespoon fresh herbs (e.g., chives, parsley)
- 1 teaspoon olive oil
- Salt and pepper to taste

Preparation:

1. In a pan, sauté mushrooms in olive oil until golden.
2. Whisk eggs, pour into the pan, and scramble.
3. Stir in fresh herbs and season to taste.

Servings: 1 | Nutritional Value (per serving):
Calories: 180, Protein: 14g, Fiber: 2g, Carbs: 5g, Fat: 12g | Cooking Time: 8 minutes

13. Peanut Butter Banana Toast

Ingredients:

- 1 slice whole grain bread
- 2 tablespoons peanut butter (unsweetened)
- 1/2 banana, sliced
- Cinnamon for garnish

Preparation:

1. Toast the bread slice.
2. Spread peanut butter on the toast and top with banana slices.
3. Sprinkle with cinnamon.

Servings: 1 | Nutritional Value (per serving): Calories: 280, Protein: 9g, Fiber: 6g, Carbs: 35g, Fat: 12g | Preparation Time: 5 minutes

14. Cranberry Walnut Overnight Oats

Ingredients:

- 1/2 cup rolled oats
- 1/2 cup almond milk (unsweetened)
- 1 tablespoon dried cranberries
- 1 tablespoon chopped walnuts
- 1/2 teaspoon vanilla extract

Preparation:

1. Mix rolled oats, almond milk, cranberries, walnuts, and vanilla extract in a jar. Refrigerate overnight.
2. Stir well before serving.

Servings: 1 | Nutritional Value (per serving): Calories: 270, Protein: 8g, Fiber: 6g, Carbs: 40g, Fat: 10g | Preparation Time: 5 minutes (plus overnight refrigeration)

15. Salmon and Dill Cream Cheese Bagel

Ingredients:

- 1 whole grain bagel, toasted
- 2 tablespoons light cream cheese
- 2 ounces smoked salmon
- Fresh dill for garnish

Preparation:

1. Spread cream cheese on the toasted bagel.
2. Layer with smoked salmon and garnish with fresh dill.

Servings: 1 | Nutritional Value (per serving): Calories: 290, Protein: 20g, Fiber: 5g, Carbs: 35g, Fat: 10g | Preparation Time: 10 minutes

Please note that these recipes provide estimated nutritional values and cooking times.

LUNCH RECIPES:

1. Grilled Lemon Herb Chicken Salad

Ingredients:

- 4 ounces grilled chicken breast, sliced
- 2 cups mixed salad greens
- 1/4 cup cherry tomatoes, halved
- 1/4 cucumber, sliced
- 1 tablespoon olive oil
- Lemon juice, salt, and pepper to taste

Preparation:

1. Combine salad greens, cherry tomatoes, and cucumber in a bowl.
2. Top with grilled chicken slices.
3. Drizzle with olive oil, lemon juice, and season with salt and pepper.

Servings: 1 | Nutritional Value (per serving): Calories: 250, Protein: 25g, Fiber: 5g, Carbs: 10g, Fat: 12g | Cooking Time: 15 minutes

2. Vegetarian Quinoa and Black Bean Bowl

Ingredients:

- 1/2 cup cooked quinoa
- 1/2 cup black beans (canned, rinsed)
- 1/2 cup bell peppers, diced
- 1/4 cup red onion, finely chopped
- 2 tablespoons cilantro, chopped
- 1 tablespoon lime juice
- 1 teaspoon olive oil

Preparation:

1. In a bowl, mix quinoa, black beans, bell peppers, red onion, and cilantro.
2. Drizzle with olive oil and lime juice, toss well, and serve.

Servings: 1 | Nutritional Value (per serving): Calories: 280, Protein: 12g, Fiber: 10g, Carbs: 45g, Fat: 7g | Cooking Time: 20 minutes

3. Salmon and Asparagus Foil Pack

Ingredients:

- 4 ounces salmon fillet
- 1/2 cup asparagus spears
- 1 tablespoon lemon juice
- 1 teaspoon dill
- Salt and pepper to taste

Preparation:

1. Place salmon and asparagus on a foil sheet.
2. Drizzle with lemon juice, sprinkle with dill, salt, and pepper.
3. Seal the foil and bake in the oven at 400°F (200°C) for 20 minutes.

Servings: 1 | Nutritional Value (per serving): Calories: 260, Protein: 25g, Fiber: 4g, Carbs: 10g, Fat: 14g | Cooking Time: 20 minutes

4. Mediterranean Chickpea Salad

Ingredients:

- 1 cup canned chickpeas, drained and rinsed
- 1/2 cup cherry tomatoes, halved
- 1/4 cup cucumber, diced
- 2 tablespoons feta cheese, crumbled
- 1 tablespoon olive oil
- Fresh basil, salt, and pepper to taste

Preparation:

1. Combine chickpeas, cherry tomatoes, cucumber, and feta in a bowl.
2. Drizzle with olive oil, add fresh basil, salt, and pepper. Toss and serve.

Servings: 1 | Nutritional Value (per serving): Calories: 280, Protein: 12g, Fiber: 8g, Carbs: 35g, Fat: 12g | Preparation Time: 10 minutes

5. Turkey and Vegetable Stir-Fry

Ingredients:

- 4 ounces lean ground turkey
- 1 cup broccoli florets
- 1/2 cup bell peppers, sliced
- 1/4 cup carrots, julienned
- 2 tablespoons low-sodium soy sauce
- 1 teaspoon ginger, minced
- 1 clove garlic, minced

Preparation:

1. In a pan, cook ground turkey until browned.
2. Add broccoli, bell peppers, carrots, ginger, and garlic. Stir-fry until vegetables are tender.
3. Add soy sauce, stir well, and serve.

Servings: 1 | Nutritional Value (per serving): Calories: 280, Protein: 26g, Fiber: 6g, Carbs: 20g, Fat: 10g | Cooking Time: 15 minutes

6. Eggplant and Tomato Stew

Ingredients:

- 1 cup eggplant, diced
- 1/2 cup cherry tomatoes, halved
- 1/4 cup onion, chopped
- 1 clove garlic, minced
- 1 tablespoon olive oil
- 1 teaspoon dried oregano
- Salt and pepper to taste

Preparation:

1. Sauté onion and garlic in olive oil until softened.
2. Add eggplant, tomatoes, oregano, salt, and pepper. Simmer until eggplant is tender.
3. Serve warm.

Servings: 1 | Nutritional Value (per serving): Calories: 220, Protein: 5g, Fiber: 10g, Carbs: 30g, Fat: 9g | Cooking Time: 20 minutes

7. Shrimp and Avocado Lettuce Wraps

Ingredients:

- 4 ounces shrimp, cooked and peeled
- 1/2 avocado, sliced
- 4 large lettuce leaves
- 1/4 cup cucumber, julienned
- 1 tablespoon cilantro, chopped
- 1 tablespoon lime juice

Preparation:

1. Arrange shrimp, avocado, cucumber, and cilantro on lettuce leaves.
2. Drizzle with lime juice and fold to create wraps.

Servings: 1 | Nutritional Value (per serving): Calories: 250, Protein: 20g, Fiber: 8g, Carbs: 15g, Fat: 14g | Preparation Time: 10 minutes

8. Stuffed Bell Peppers with Quinoa and Black Beans

Ingredients:

- 2 bell peppers, halved
- 1/2 cup cooked quinoa
- 1/2 cup black beans (canned, rinsed)
- 1/4 cup corn kernels
- 1/4 cup salsa (low-sodium)
- 1/4 cup shredded low-fat cheese

Preparation:

1. Preheat oven to 375°F (190°C).
2. Mix quinoa, black beans, corn, and salsa in a bowl.
3. Stuff bell pepper halves with the mixture, top with shredded cheese, and bake for 20-25 minutes.

Servings: 1 | Nutritional Value (per serving): Calories: 300, Protein: 15g, Fiber: 10g, Carbs: 40g, Fat: 8g | Cooking Time: 25 minutes

9. Chicken and Vegetable Skewers

Ingredients:

- 4 ounces chicken breast, cubed
- 1/2 cup bell peppers, sliced
- 1/2 cup zucchini, sliced
- 1 tablespoon olive oil
- 1 teaspoon rosemary, chopped
- Salt and pepper to taste

Preparation:

1. Thread chicken, bell peppers, and zucchini onto skewers.
2. Mix olive oil, rosemary, salt, and pepper. Brush over skewers.
3. Grill or bake for 15-20 minutes until chicken is cooked.

Servings: 1 | Nutritional Value (per serving):
Calories: 280, Protein: 25g, Fiber: 6g, Carbs: 15g, Fat: 14g | Cooking Time: 20 minutes

10. Cauliflower and Broccoli Rice Bowl

Ingredients:

- 1 cup cauliflower rice
- 1/2 cup broccoli florets
- 1/4 cup carrots, shredded
- 2 tablespoons low-sodium soy sauce
- 1 tablespoon sesame oil
- 1 green onion, chopped

Preparation:

1. In a pan, sauté cauliflower rice, broccoli, and carrots.
2. Add soy sauce and sesame oil. Stir-fry until vegetables are tender.
3. Top with chopped green onions and serve.

Servings: 1 | Nutritional Value (per serving): Calories: 180, Protein: 6g, Fiber: 8g, Carbs: 20g, Fat: 9g | Cooking Time: 15 minutes

11. Tomato Basil Lentil Soup

Ingredients:

- 1/2 cup dry lentils, rinsed
- 1 cup tomatoes, diced
- 1/4 cup onion, chopped
- 1 clove garlic, minced
- 1 tablespoon olive oil
- 1 teaspoon dried basil
- Salt and pepper to taste

Preparation:

1. In a pot, sauté onion and garlic in olive oil until softened.
2. Add lentils, tomatoes, basil, salt, and pepper. Cover with water and simmer until lentils are cooked.

Servings: 2 | Nutritional Value (per serving): Calories: 220, Protein: 12g, Fiber: 12g, Carbs: 30g, Fat: 7g | Cooking Time: 30 minutes

12. Tuna and White Bean Salad

Ingredients:

- 1/2 cup canned white beans, drained and rinsed
- 2 ounces canned tuna, drained
- 1/4 cup cherry tomatoes, halved
- 1 tablespoon red onion, finely chopped
- 1 tablespoon balsamic vinaigrette

Preparation:

1. Combine white beans, tuna, cherry tomatoes, and red onion in a bowl.
2. Drizzle with balsamic vinaigrette, toss, and serve.

Servings: 1 | Nutritional Value (per serving): Calories: 250, Protein: 20g, Fiber: 7g, Carbs: 25g, Fat: 9g | Preparation Time: 10 minutes

13. Cabbage and Turkey Sauté

Ingredients:

- 4 ounces ground turkey
- 1 cup cabbage, shredded
- 1/2 cup bell peppers, sliced
- 1/4 cup onion, sliced
- 1 tablespoon olive oil
- 1 teaspoon paprika
- Salt and pepper to taste

Preparation:

1. In a pan, cook ground turkey until browned.
2. Add cabbage, bell peppers, onion, olive oil, paprika, salt, and pepper. Sauté until vegetables are tender.

Servings: 1 | Nutritional Value (per serving): Calories: 280, Protein: 22g, Fiber: 7g, Carbs: 15g, Fat: 15g | Cooking Time: 15 minutes

14. Sweet Potato and Black Bean Quesadilla

Ingredients:

- 1 small sweet potato, cooked and mashed
- 1/2 cup black beans (canned, rinsed)
- 1 whole wheat tortilla
- 1/4 cup shredded low-fat cheese
- 1 tablespoon salsa (low-sodium)

Preparation:

1. Spread sweet potato on one half of the tortilla.
2. Top with black beans, shredded cheese, and salsa.
3. Fold the tortilla in half and cook on a griddle until cheese melts.

Servings: 1 | Nutritional Value (per serving): Calories: 300, Protein: 15g, Fiber: 10g, Carbs: 40g, Fat: 10g | Cooking Time: 10 minutes

15. Sesame Ginger Chicken Bowl

Ingredients:

- 4 ounces grilled chicken breast, sliced
- 1/2 cup broccoli, steamed
- 1/4 cup snap peas, sliced
- 1/2 cup brown rice, cooked
- 1 tablespoon low-sodium soy sauce
- 1 teaspoon sesame oil
- 1 teaspoon ginger, grated

Preparation:

1. Combine grilled chicken, steamed broccoli, snap peas, and brown rice in a bowl.
2. Drizzle with soy sauce, sesame oil, and sprinkle with grated ginger. Toss and serve.

Servings: 1 | Nutritional Value (per serving): Calories: 320, Protein: 30g, Fiber: 6g, Carbs: 40g, Fat: 7g | Cooking Time: 20 minutes

DINNER RECIPES:

1. Baked Lemon Herb Salmon

Ingredients:

- 1 salmon fillet
- 1 tablespoon lemon juice
- 1 teaspoon dried herbs (such as thyme or dill)
- 1 teaspoon olive oil
- Salt and pepper to taste

Preparation:

1. Preheat oven to 400°F (200°C).
2. Place the salmon on a baking sheet.
3. Drizzle with lemon juice and olive oil, sprinkle with dried herbs, salt, and pepper.
4. Bake for 15-20 minutes or until the salmon is cooked through.

Servings: 1 | Nutritional Value (per serving): Calories: 250, Protein: 25g, Fiber: 1g, Carbs: 0g, Fat: 16g | Cooking Time: 20 minutes

2. Vegetarian Lentil Soup

Ingredients:

- 1/2 cup dry lentils, rinsed
- 1 carrot, diced
- 1 celery stalk, chopped
- 1/4 cup onion, finely chopped
- 1 clove garlic, minced
- 4 cups low-sodium vegetable broth
- 1 teaspoon olive oil
- 1 teaspoon cumin
- Salt and pepper to taste

Preparation:

1. In a pot, sauté onion and garlic in olive oil until softened.
2. Add lentils, carrot, celery, cumin, salt, and pepper. Pour in vegetable broth.
3. Simmer for 25-30 minutes or until lentils are tender.

Servings: 2 | Nutritional Value (per serving): Calories: 200, Protein: 15g, Fiber: 10g, Carbs: 30g, Fat: 3g | Cooking Time: 30 minutes

3. Grilled Turkey and Vegetable Kebabs

Ingredients:

- 4 ounces turkey breast, cubed
- 1/2 bell pepper, cut into chunks
- 1/2 zucchini, sliced
- Cherry tomatoes
- 1 tablespoon olive oil
- 1 teaspoon Italian seasoning
- Salt and pepper to taste

Preparation:

1. Preheat the grill.
2. Thread turkey, bell pepper, zucchini, and tomatoes onto skewers.
3. Brush with olive oil, sprinkle with Italian seasoning, salt, and pepper.
4. Grill for 10-15 minutes, turning occasionally, until turkey is cooked.

Servings: 1 | Nutritional Value (per serving): Calories: 280, Protein: 25g, Fiber: 5g, Carbs: 10g, Fat: 15g | Cooking Time: 15 minutes

4. Eggplant and Chickpea Curry

Ingredients:

- 1 cup eggplant, diced
- 1/2 cup canned chickpeas, drained and rinsed
- 1/2 cup tomatoes, diced
- 1/4 cup onion, chopped
- 1 clove garlic, minced
- 1 tablespoon olive oil
- 1 teaspoon curry powder
- Salt and pepper to taste

Preparation:

1. Sauté onion and garlic in olive oil until softened.
2. Add eggplant, chickpeas, tomatoes, curry powder, salt, and pepper.
3. Cook for 20-25 minutes or until eggplant is tender.

Servings: 2 | Nutritional Value (per serving): Calories: 220, Protein: 8g, Fiber: 12g, Carbs: 30g, Fat: 8g | Cooking Time: 25 minutes

5. Shrimp and Quinoa Stir-Fry

Ingredients:

- 4 ounces shrimp, peeled and deveined
- 1/2 cup cooked quinoa
- 1/2 cup broccoli florets
- 1/4 cup bell peppers, sliced
- 1 tablespoon low-sodium soy sauce
- 1 teaspoon sesame oil
- 1 teaspoon ginger, minced

Preparation:

1. In a pan, stir-fry shrimp, broccoli, and bell peppers until shrimp is pink.
2. Add cooked quinoa, soy sauce, sesame oil, and ginger.
3. Cook for an additional 5 minutes, stirring continuously.

Servings: 1 | Nutritional Value (per serving): Calories: 290, Protein: 25g, Fiber: 6g, Carbs: 35g, Fat: 8g | Cooking Time: 15 minutes

6. Baked Chicken and Vegetable Casserole

Ingredients:

- 1 chicken thigh, boneless and skinless
- 1/2 cup sweet potatoes, diced
- 1/2 cup Brussels sprouts, halved
- 1/4 cup red onion, sliced
- 1 tablespoon olive oil
- 1 teaspoon rosemary, chopped
- Salt and pepper to taste

Preparation:

1. Preheat oven to 375°F (190°C).
2. Place chicken, sweet potatoes, Brussels sprouts, and red onion in a baking dish.
3. Drizzle with olive oil, sprinkle with rosemary, salt, and pepper.
4. Bake for 30-35 minutes or until chicken is cooked through.

Servings: 1 | Nutritional Value (per serving):
Calories: 300, Protein: 20g, Fiber: 7g, Carbs: 25g, Fat: 15g | Cooking Time: 35 minutes

7. Salmon and Asparagus Stir-Fry

Ingredients:

- 4 ounces salmon fillet, cubed
- 1/2 cup asparagus, sliced
- 1/4 cup carrots, julienned
- 1/4 cup snow peas
- 1 tablespoon low-sodium soy sauce
- 1 teaspoon honey
- 1 teaspoon sesame oil

Preparation:

1. In a wok, stir-fry salmon, asparagus, carrots, and snow peas until salmon is cooked.
2. In a small bowl, mix soy sauce, honey, and sesame oil. Pour over the stir-fry and toss.
3. Cook for an additional 2-3 minutes.

Servings: 1 | Nutritional Value (per serving): Calories: 280, Protein: 25g, Fiber: 6g, Carbs: 15g, Fat: 14g | Cooking Time: 10 minutes

8. Quinoa and Vegetable Stuffed Peppers

Ingredients:

- 2 bell peppers, halved
- 1/2 cup cooked quinoa
- 1/2 cup black beans (canned, rinsed)
- 1/4 cup corn kernels
- 1/4 cup salsa (low-sodium)
- 1/4 cup shredded low-fat cheese

Preparation:

1. Preheat oven to 375°F (190°C).
2. Mix quinoa, black beans, corn, and salsa in a bowl.
3. Stuff bell pepper halves with the mixture, top with shredded cheese, and bake for 20-25 minutes.

Servings: 1 | Nutritional Value (per serving): Calories: 300, Protein: 15g, Fiber: 10g, Carbs: 40g, Fat: 8g | Cooking Time: 25 minutes

9. Miso Glazed Tofu with Steamed Broccoli

Ingredients:

- 1/2 cup firm tofu, cubed
- 1 cup broccoli florets
- 1 tablespoon miso paste
- 1 tablespoon low-sodium soy sauce
- 1 teaspoon sesame oil
- 1 teaspoon rice vinegar

Preparation:

1. Steam broccoli until tender.
2. In a pan, sauté tofu until golden.
3. In a bowl, mix miso paste, soy sauce, sesame oil, and rice vinegar. Pour over tofu.
4. Serve tofu over steamed broccoli.

Servings: 1 | Nutritional Value (per serving): Calories: 220, Protein: 15g, Fiber: 8g, Carbs: 20g, Fat: 12g | Cooking Time: 15 minutes

10. Zucchini Noodles with Tomato Basil Sauce

Ingredients:

- 1 medium zucchini, spiralized
- 1/2 cup cherry tomatoes, halved
- 1/4 cup onion, finely chopped
- 1 clove garlic, minced
- 2 tablespoons tomato sauce (low-sodium)
- 1 tablespoon olive oil
- Fresh basil, salt, and pepper to taste

Preparation:

1. In a pan, sauté onion and garlic in olive oil until softened.
2. Add zucchini noodles, cherry tomatoes, and tomato sauce. Cook for 5-7 minutes.
3. Season with salt, pepper, and garnish with fresh basil.

Servings: 1 | Nutritional Value (per serving):
Calories: 180, Protein: 6g, Fiber: 5g, Carbs: 20g, Fat: 10g | Cooking Time: 10 minutes

11. Cauliflower Pizza with Turkey and Veggies

Ingredients:

- 1 cup cauliflower rice
- 1/4 cup egg whites
- 2 tablespoons almond flour
- 1/2 cup ground turkey, cooked
- 1/4 cup bell peppers, diced
- 1/4 cup tomatoes, diced
- 1/4 cup low-sodium pizza sauce
- 1/4 cup shredded low-fat cheese

Preparation:

1. Preheat oven to 425°F (220°C).
2. Mix cauliflower rice, egg whites, and almond flour to form a crust. Bake for 15 minutes.
3. Spread pizza sauce on the crust, top with turkey, bell peppers, tomatoes, and cheese.
4. Bake for an additional 10-12 minutes or until the cheese is melted.

Servings: 1 | Nutritional Value (per serving): Calories: 280, Protein: 25g, Fiber: 8g, Carbs: 20g, Fat: 15g | Cooking Time: 25 minutes

12. Stir-Fried Ginger Sesame Beef

Ingredients:

- 4 ounces lean beef, thinly sliced
- 1/2 cup broccoli florets
- 1/4 cup snap peas
- 1/4 cup carrots, julienned
- 1 tablespoon low-sodium soy sauce
- 1 tablespoon sesame oil
- 1 teaspoon ginger, minced

Preparation:

1. In a wok, stir-fry beef, broccoli, snap peas, and carrots until beef is cooked.
2. In a small bowl, mix soy sauce, sesame oil, and ginger. Pour over the stir-fry and toss.
3. Cook for an additional 2-3 minutes.

Servings: 1 | Nutritional Value (per serving): Calories: 290, Protein: 25g, Fiber: 6g, Carbs: 15g, Fat: 14g | Cooking Time: 10 minutes

13. Spaghetti Squash with Tomato and Basil Sauce

Ingredients:

- 1/2 medium spaghetti squash, roasted
- 1/2 cup cherry tomatoes, halved
- 1/4 cup onion, finely chopped
- 1 clove garlic, minced
- 2 tablespoons tomato sauce (low-sodium)
- 1 tablespoon olive oil
- Fresh basil, salt, and pepper to taste

Preparation:

1. In a pan, sauté onion and garlic in olive oil until softened.
2. Add spaghetti squash, cherry tomatoes, and tomato sauce. Cook for 5-7 minutes.
3. Season with salt, pepper, and garnish with fresh basil.

Servings: 1 | Nutritional Value (per serving): Calories: 200, Protein: 6g, Fiber: 8g, Carbs: 25g, Fat: 10g | Cooking Time: 10 minutes

SNACK AND DESSERT RECIPES:

Greek Yogurt and Berry Parfait

Ingredients:

- 1/2 cup Greek yogurt (unsweetened)
- 1/4 cup mixed berries (blueberries, strawberries)
- 1 tablespoon chopped almonds
- 1/2 teaspoon honey (optional)

Preparation:

1. In a glass, layer Greek yogurt, mixed berries, and chopped almonds.
2. Drizzle with honey if desired.

Servings: 1 | Nutritional Value (per serving): Calories: 150, Protein: 10g, Fiber: 3g, Carbs: 15g, Fat: 7g | Preparation Time: 5 minutes

Vegetable Sticks with Hummus

Ingredients:

1. 1/2 cup carrot and cucumber sticks
2. 2 tablespoons hummus (low-sodium)

Preparation:

1. Arrange carrot and cucumber sticks on a plate.
2. Serve with hummus for dipping.

Servings: 1 | Nutritional Value (per serving): Calories: 80, Protein: 3g, Fiber: 5g, Carbs: 12g, Fat: 4g | Preparation Time: 5 minutes

Hard-Boiled Egg and Avocado

Ingredients:

- 1 hard-boiled egg
- 1/2 avocado, sliced
- Sprinkle of black pepper

Preparation:

1. Slice the hard-boiled egg and arrange with avocado slices.
2. Sprinkle with black pepper.

Servings: 1 | Nutritional Value (per serving): Calories: 180, Protein: 7g, Fiber: 7g, Carbs: 9g, Fat: 13g | Preparation Time: 7 minutes

Cottage Cheese and Pineapple Cup

Ingredients:

- 1/2 cup low-fat cottage cheese
- 1/2 cup fresh pineapple chunks

Preparation:

1. Combine cottage cheese and fresh pineapple in a cup.

Servings: 1 | Nutritional Value (per serving): Calories: 120, Protein: 14g, Fiber: 1g, Carbs: 16g, Fat: 2g | Preparation Time: 3 minutes

Almond Butter and Banana Rice Cake

Ingredients:

- 1 rice cake (low-sodium)
- 1 tablespoon almond butter (unsweetened)
- 1/2 banana, sliced

Preparation:

1. Spread almond butter on the rice cake.
2. Top with banana slices.

Servings: 1 | Nutritional Value (per serving): Calories: 180, Protein: 4g, Fiber: 3g, Carbs: 25g, Fat: 8g | Preparation Time: 5 minutes

Chia Seed Pudding with Berries

Ingredients:

- 2 tablespoons chia seeds
- 1/2 cup almond milk (unsweetened)
- 1/2 teaspoon vanilla extract
- 1/4 cup mixed berries

Preparation:

1. Mix chia seeds, almond milk, and vanilla extract in a jar. Refrigerate overnight.
2. Top with mixed berries before serving.

Servings: 1 | Nutritional Value (per serving): Calories: 150, Protein: 4g, Fiber: 8g, Carbs: 15g, Fat: 8g | Preparation Time: 5 minutes (plus overnight refrigeration)

Baked Apple with Cinnamon

Ingredients:

- 1 small apple, cored and sliced
- 1/2 teaspoon cinnamon
- 1 tablespoon chopped walnuts (optional)

Preparation:

1. Place apple slices on a baking sheet.
2. Sprinkle with cinnamon and bake at 350°F (175°C) for 15 minutes.
3. Top with chopped walnuts if desired.

Servings: 1 | Nutritional Value (per serving): Calories: 90, Protein: 1g, Fiber: 5g, Carbs: 20g, Fat: 2g | Cooking Time: 15 minutes

Frozen Yogurt Berry Bites

Ingredients:

- 1/2 cup Greek yogurt (unsweetened)
- 1/4 cup mixed berries (blueberries, raspberries)
- 1 teaspoon honey (optional)

Preparation:

1. Mix Greek yogurt and berries in a bowl.
2. Spoon into small silicone molds and freeze until firm.
3. Pop out the yogurt bites and drizzle with honey if desired.

Servings: 1 | Nutritional Value (per serving): Calories: 70, Protein: 5g, Fiber: 1g, Carbs: 10g, Fat: 1g | Preparation Time: 10 minutes (plus freezing time)

Avocado Chocolate Mousse

Ingredients:

- 1 ripe avocado
- 2 tablespoons cocoa powder (unsweetened)
- 2 tablespoons honey
- 1/2 teaspoon vanilla extract

Preparation:

1. Blend avocado, cocoa powder, honey, and vanilla extract until smooth.
2. Chill in the refrigerator before serving.

Servings: 1 | Nutritional Value (per serving): Calories: 200, Protein: 3g, Fiber: 7g, Carbs: 20g, Fat: 15g | Preparation Time: 5 minutes

Peach and Almond Yogurt Parfait

Ingredients:

- 1/2 cup low-fat vanilla yogurt
- 1 peach, sliced
- 1 tablespoon sliced almonds

Preparation:

1. In a glass, layer vanilla yogurt, sliced peaches, and almonds.

Servings: 1 | Nutritional Value (per serving): Calories: 160, Protein: 6g, Fiber: 2g, Carbs: 30g, Fat: 3g | Preparation Time: 5 minutes

Coconut Chia Mango Sorbet

Ingredients:

- 1/2 cup frozen mango chunks
- 2 tablespoons coconut milk (unsweetened)
- 1 tablespoon chia seeds
- 1 teaspoon lime juice

Preparation:

1. Blend frozen mango, coconut milk, chia seeds, and lime juice until smooth.
2. Freeze for 2 hours before serving.

Servings: 1 | Nutritional Value (per serving): Calories: 120, Protein: 3g, Fiber: 7g, Carbs: 20g, Fat: 5g | Preparation Time: 10 minutes (plus freezing time)

Berry and Walnut Oat Bars

Ingredients:

- 1/2 cup rolled oats
- 1/4 cup mixed berries (strawberries, blueberries)
- 1/4 cup chopped walnuts
- 1 tablespoon honey

Preparation:

1. Mix rolled oats, berries, walnuts, and honey in a bowl.
2. Press into a small baking dish and refrigerate until firm. Cut into bars.

Servings: 1 | Nutritional Value (per serving): Calories: 180, Protein: 4g, Fiber: 5g, Carbs: 25g, Fat: 8g | Preparation Time: 10 minutes (plus refrigeration time)

Pumpkin Pie Smoothie

Ingredients:

- 1/2 cup canned pumpkin (unsweetened)
- 1/2 banana
- 1/2 cup almond milk (unsweetened)
- 1/2 teaspoon pumpkin pie spice
- Ice cubes

Preparation:

1. Blend pumpkin, banana, almond milk, pumpkin pie spice, and ice cubes until smooth.

Servings: 1 | Nutritional Value (per serving): Calories: 120, Protein: 2g, Fiber: 6g, Carbs: 30g, Fat: 1g | Preparation Time: 5 minutes

Raspberry Coconut Chia Popsicles

Ingredients:

- 1/2 cup raspberries
- 1/2 cup coconut water
- 1 tablespoon chia seeds
- 1 teaspoon honey

Preparation:

1. Blend raspberries, coconut water, chia seeds, and honey until smooth.
2. Pour into popsicle molds and freeze until solid.

Servings: 1 | Nutritional Value (per serving): Calories: 80, Protein: 2g, Fiber: 7g, Carbs: 15g, Fat: 3g | Preparation Time: 10 minutes (plus freezing time)

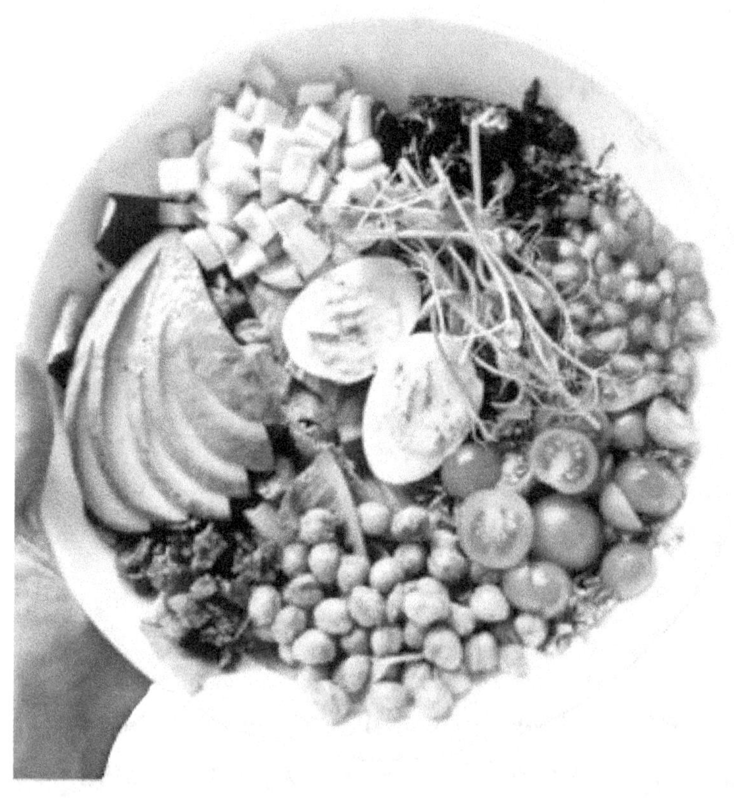

CONCLUSION:

In the Stage 3 Kidney Disease Diet Cookbook for Seniors, I want to emphasize the incredible potential for positive change that lies within the simple act of choosing the right foods. We've explored a myriad of flavors and textures, crafting recipes that dance in harmony with the intricate needs of those managing stage 3 kidney disease, diabetes, or heart concerns.

Remember, this isn't just a collection of recipes; it's a roadmap to a healthier, more vibrant life. Each dish is a step toward not merely managing but thriving in the face of health challenges. As a seasoned nutritionist, I've witnessed firsthand the profound impact that conscious nutrition can have on the trajectory of one's well-being.

The journey toward better health may seem daunting, but it begins with small, intentional steps.

The recipes within these pages aren't just sustenance for the body; they are an invitation to a new way of living. A life where you savor each bite, knowing that it contributes not only to your enjoyment but also to your vitality.

So, I invite you to embark on this culinary adventure. Let these recipes be your companions on the path to wellness. Picture the future where your health story unfolds with resilience, where each meal is a declaration of self-care, and where you savor not just the flavors but the victories of a well-nourished life.

In the words of an ancient proverb, **"The groundwork of all happiness is health."** Today, you hold in your hands not just a cookbook but a key to unlock a happier, healthier chapter of your life. Let the nourishment within these pages be the catalyst for your well-being. May you savor not only the delectable tastes but also the joy of taking charge of your health. Here's to a future of delicious possibilities and a life well-lived!

MEAL PLANNER

DATE:

	BREAKFAST	LUNCH	DINNER	SHOPPING LIST
MON				
TUES				
WED				
THURS				
FRI				
SAT				
SUN				

MEAL PLANNER

DATE:

	BREAKFAST	LUNCH	DINNER	SHOPPING LIST
MON				
TUES				
WED				
THURS				
FRI				
SAT				
SUN				

MEAL PLANNER

DATE:

	BREAKFAST	LUNCH	DINNER	SHOPPING LIST
MON				
TUES				
WED				
THURS				
FRI				
SAT				
SUN				

MEAL PLANNER

DATE:

	BREAKFAST	LUNCH	DINNER	SHOPPING LIST
MON				
TUES				
WED				
THURS				
FRI				
SAT				
SUN				

MEAL PLANNER

DATE:

	BREAKFAST	LUNCH	DINNER	SHOPPING LIST
MON				
TUES				
WED				
THURS				
FRI				
SAT				
SUN				

MEAL PLANNER

DATE:

	BREAKFAST	LUNCH	DINNER	SHOPPING LIST
MON				
TUES				
WED				
THURS				
FRI				
SAT				
SUN				

MEAL PLANNER

DATE:

	BREAKFAST	LUNCH	DINNER	SHOPPING LIST
MON				
TUES				
WED				
THURS				
FRI				
SAT				
SUN				

MEAL PLANNER

DATE:

	BREAKFAST	LUNCH	DINNER	SHOPPING LIST
MON				
TUES				
WED				
THURS				
FRI				
SAT				
SUN				

MEAL PLANNER

DATE:

	BREAKFAST	LUNCH	DINNER	SHOPPING LIST
MON				
TUES				
WED				
THURS				
FRI				
SAT				
SUN				

MEAL PLANNER

DATE:

	BREAKFAST	LUNCH	DINNER	SHOPPING LIST
MON				
TUES				
WED				
THURS				
FRI				
SAT				
SUN				

MEAL PLANNER

DATE:

	BREAKFAST	LUNCH	DINNER	SHOPPING LIST
MON				
TUES				
WED				
THURS				
FRI				
SAT				
SUN				

MEAL PLANNER

DATE:

	BREAKFAST	LUNCH	DINNER	SHOPPING LIST
MON				
TUES				
WED				
THURS				
FRI				
SAT				
SUN				

MEAL PLANNER

DATE:

	BREAKFAST	LUNCH	DINNER	SHOPPING LIST
MON				
TUES				
WED				
THURS				
FRI				
SAT				
SUN				

MEAL PLANNER

DATE:

	BREAKFAST	LUNCH	DINNER	SHOPPING LIST
MON				
TUES				
WED				
THURS				
FRI				
SAT				
SUN				

www.ingramcontent.com/pod-product-compliance
Lightning Source LLC
Chambersburg PA
CBHW070902260726

48661CB00004B/1561